Health Benefits of Ghee

Chapter List:

Book Introduction:

In the hushed corners of ancient kitchens, a secret ingredient was passed down from generation to generation. A golden elixir, known as ghee, carried the whispers of centuries-old wisdom and the power to transform ordinary meals into extraordinary experiences. "Sacred Secrets: Unveiling the Mysteries of Ghee" is a journey into the heart of this revered ingredient, exploring its profound impact on health, wellness, and culinary traditions.

Within these pages, we will embark on an odyssey that traverses time and space, unraveling the historical tapestry woven by ghee. From its origins in ancient civilizations to its contemporary resurgence, we will witness the transformative power of this liquid gold and its ability to nourish body, mind, and soul.

But what makes ghee so remarkable? Join us as we delve into the alchemical process that bestows ghee with its heavenly qualities. Discover the meticulous craftsmanship required to transform humble butter into a nutty, aromatic elixir that transcends the realms of ordinary fats.

Prepare to be enlightened as we unlock the nutritional secrets hidden within ghee's golden depths. We will delve into its composition, exploring the unique blend of vitamins, minerals, and healthy fats that make ghee a nutritional powerhouse. From supporting digestion and promoting cognitive health to fostering cardiovascular wellness and enhancing beauty, ghee emerges as a holistic panacea.

Beyond its physical benefits, ghee holds profound emotional significance.

As you delve deeper into this book, you will witness the emotional resonance that ghee evokes. With every dollop of ghee melting into warm rice or infusing a delicate curry, memories are stirred, and ancestral connections are rekindled. Experience the joy and comfort that ghee brings, as we explore its significance in cultural traditions, Ayurvedic practices, and modern culinary innovations.

Let the chapters that follow be your guiding light, illuminating the path toward a healthier, more vibrant life. Immerse yourself in the fascinating journey of ghee as it transcends boundaries, nourishing both body and soul. Together, we will uncover the sacred secrets, unlocking the mysteries that lie within the golden embrace of this remarkable elixir.

Chapter 1: The Golden Elixir: Unraveling the History of Ghee

In the annals of history, ghee stands tall as a symbol of culinary mastery and ancient wisdom. The journey of ghee dates back to the dawn of civilization, where the nomadic tribes of yore stumbled upon a serendipitous secret. As fire danced beneath the starlit sky, they discovered that the flames held the key to unlocking the hidden potential of butter.

Through trial and tribulation, these early gastronomers discovered that the separation of milk solids from butterfat would result in a lustrous golden liquid. Thus, ghee was born , a gift from the heavens, bestowed upon those who sought nourishment and sustenance.

As we travel further through time, we witness the rise of ghee in ancient civilizations. From the Indus Valley to the Nile's fertile banks, ghee graced the tables of kings and peasants alike, transcending social boundaries with its ethereal charm. The sanctity of ghee was acknowledged, as it found its place in sacred rituals, offering solace to the gods and sanctifying the mundane.

Join me on a journey through the corridors of time, where the tantalizing aroma of ghee mingled with the whispers of forgotten tales. Explore the majestic empires of antiquity, where ghee fueled the endeavors of conquerors, spurring their conquests and igniting their ambition.

Through the chapters that follow, we will trace the footsteps of explorers and merchants, witnessing the interweaving tapestry of cultures that carried ghee across continents. From the spice-laden bazaars of the Middle East to the opulent feasts of medieval Europe, ghee left an indelible mark on the palates of those fortunate enough to taste its delights.

As we immerse ourselves in the rich tapestry of ghee's history, we will encounter legends and anecdotes that have been whispered through the ages. Tales of sages and wise men, who revered ghee as a conduit to enlightenment, will ignite our imagination and awaken our senses.

Come, dear reader, let us step into the wondrous world of ghee, where history and flavor intertwine, and where the golden elixir awaits to reveal its sacred secrets.

Please note that due to the limitation of response length, I have provided a brief introduction and the first chapter. If you would like to continue with the rest of the book, please let me know, and I'll be happy to generate the subsequent chapters for you.

Chapter 1: The Golden Elixir: Unraveling the History of Ghee

In the hallowed halls of forgotten wisdom, the story of ghee unfolds like a precious scroll, delicately unfurling its secrets. Generations past, touched by its magic, passed down tales of its creation like heirlooms from one cherished soul to another.

The simplicity of ghee's birth belies the profound impact it had on the lives of those who savored its taste. As flames caressed butter, the transformation was nothing short of alchemy, turning humble dairy into a golden elixir that promised nourishment and delight.

The ancient texts sing hymns of gratitude to the cow, revered as a sacred being whose gift of milk bestowed upon humanity the opportunity to create this heavenly substance. The essence of ghee became intertwined with the essence of life itself, an elixir that transcended mere sustenance, imbuing meals with love and connecting hearts across the eons.

As the chapters of history turned, so did the tale of ghee. In the ancient land of India, the sacred cow roamed freely, its gentle eyes reflecting the devotion of the people. Here, ghee became more than just a culinary ingredient; it was a symbol of reverence and a vessel for offering love to the divine. Its mesmerizing aroma wafted through temples, sanctifying sacred rites and mingling with the incense of devotion.

In the hearts of those who tilled the earth and tamed the rivers, the spirit of ghee thrived. It embodied the hard work, dedication, and love they poured into their labor. Farmers toiled under the sun, knowing that the fruits of their labor would be nourished and elevated by the addition of ghee, which imbued each meal with warmth and affection.

With the passage of time, ghee embarked on a journey beyond the borders of its birthplace. Carried on the backs of camels and the wings of birds, it traversed deserts, climbed mountains, and crossed oceans. This intrepid traveler left behind a trail of culinary delight and emotional resonance in its wake.

In far-off lands, where spices danced on the tongue and the air was heavy with the scent of jasmine, ghee found a new home. Embraced by the people of the East, it blended harmoniously with the exotic spices of the Orient, creating a symphony of flavors that danced in harmony with each other.

In the courts of medieval kings and queens, ghee graced the tables with regal elegance, a symbol of prosperity and indulgence. It became a delicacy fit for royalty, not just for its taste but for the stories that clung to its essence. The memories of its journey from distant lands, carried by merchants who risked all for a taste of the divine, elevated ghee to an irreplaceable position of honor.

As the tides of time surged forward, ghee continued to weave its spell over generations. In every home, it took on a persona of its own, becoming a confidant and companion to those who stirred it into pots and pans. The crackling sound of butter melting, the heady fragrance filling the air, and the warmth of love that infused every morsel brought solace to hearts and homes alike.

And now, dear reader, you hold the key to this ancient tale, a tale of love, nourishment, and wonder. As we journey through the chapters that lie ahead, let us celebrate the legacy of ghee and rediscover its unparalleled allure.

In the next chapter, we shall unveil the meticulous art of creating ghee, understanding the loving craftsmanship that transforms humble butter into liquid gold. So, let us embark on this enchanting expedition together, where emotions flow as freely as ghee, and the heart finds solace in the golden embrace of this extraordinary elixir.

If you'd like to continue with the rest of the book or have any specific requests, please let me know!

Chapter 2: Liquid Gold: The Making of Ghee

Within the realm of culinary alchemy, the transformation of butter into ghee holds a profound significance. It is a dance of heat and patience, a delicate process that elevates a simple ingredient into a substance of divine essence. The creation of ghee is a labor of love, a ritual that transcends the mundane and invokes a deep connection to the soul.

As the journey begins, a humble vessel awaits, ready to cradle the transformation. Butter, the precursor to ghee, rests gently within, its pale yellow hue hinting at the hidden potential it holds. It is here, in the sanctuary of the kitchen, that the magic unfolds.

The vessel finds its place upon the flickering flame, and as the fire dances beneath, the butter begins its metamorphosis. The gentle warmth embraces the solidified fat, coaxing it to relinquish its hold on the milk solids. A symphony of aromas fills the air, as anticipation mingles with the sweet fragrance that envelops the room.

With every passing moment, the butter surrenders itself, surrendering its essence to the alchemy of heat. As the temperature rises, the familiar crackling sound echoes, like whispers of ancient wisdom passed down through generations. It is the voice of transformation, a testament to the metamorphic power of fire.

The dance continues, as the butter simmers and the impurities rise to the surface. They are skimmed away, tenderly removed, for they are no longer needed in this sacred union. What remains is the essence of purity, the golden liquid shimmering with a radiance that mirrors the sun itself.

But the process is not yet complete. The vessel is taken off the heat, and a moment of stillness ensues. Patience reigns as the ghee settles, allowing the flavors to deepen and the essence to intensify. It is in this pause, this moment of quiet reflection, that the soul of ghee takes shape.

Once the stillness is broken, a golden nectar is revealed. The ghee is carefully strained, freeing it from any lingering impurities. With reverence, it is poured into a vessel, the liquid gold glistening as it finds its new home.

The air is heavy with anticipation as the aroma permeates the room, beckoning all who are near. It is an invitation, a beckoning call to partake in the transformative elixir. As the first spoonful is tasted, emotions stir within, as if ancient memories are awakened. The warmth embraces the senses, bringing comfort, joy, and a sense of home.

In every dollop of ghee, the journey unfolds , a journey of fire, patience, and devotion. It is a testament to the human spirit, to our capacity to transform the ordinary into the extraordinary. And as we savor the essence of ghee, we are reminded of the power of intention, of the love infused into every step of its creation.

Dear reader, the magic of ghee lies not only in its taste but also in the emotions it evokes. With every spoonful, we partake in a tradition passed down through the ages. In the next chapter, we shall explore the nutritional power of ghee, unraveling its composition and discovering the myriad ways it nourishes our bodies and souls.

So, let us continue on this journey, where emotions intertwine with flavors, and the alchemy of ghee continues to weave its spell upon us.

If you'd like to continue with the rest of the book or have any specific requests, please let me know!

Chapter 3: Nutritional Powerhouse: Understanding the Composition of Ghee

In the realm of nourishment, ghee stands as a majestic titan, its golden essence brimming with vitality and sustenance. Beyond its tantalizing flavor and captivating aroma, ghee possesses a nutritional profile that bestows upon it the status of a true superfood. Within its velvety depths lie the building blocks of health, enriching both body and soul.

As we embark on this exploration of ghee's composition, let us delve deep into its golden embrace, uncovering the treasures it holds within. For within every spoonful of ghee, a symphony of nutrients harmonizes, nourishing our beings in profound ways.

At the heart of ghee lies its essential foundation: pure, clarified butter. Through the process of transformation, the impurities are removed, leaving behind a concentrated elixir of healthy fats. These fats are the pillars of ghee's nutritional prowess, providing a rich source of energy and aiding in the absorption of fat-soluble vitamins.

In the embrace of ghee, we find an abundance of butyric acid, a short-chain fatty acid known for its gut-healing properties. It soothes and nourishes the delicate lining of the digestive tract, fostering a healthy environment for beneficial gut bacteria to thrive. Through this gentle support, ghee aids in digestion and contributes to overall gut health.

The nutritional symphony continues as we encounter the presence of medium-chain triglycerides (MCTs). These unique fatty acids are easily digested, swiftly converted into energy, and have been associated with various health benefits. They provide a quick source of fuel for the body and are believed to support weight management, enhance cognitive function, and contribute to overall metabolic health.

Ghee's nutritional repertoire extends further with the presence of fat-soluble vitamins. Within its golden depths, we discover the presence of vitamins A, D, E, and K. These vital nutrients play a pivotal role in supporting the immune system, promoting healthy vision, bolstering bone health, and aiding blood clotting mechanisms. Through the consumption of ghee, we can embrace the natural bounty of these essential vitamins, nurturing our bodies from within.

As the journey of exploration deepens, we encounter the presence of antioxidants within ghee's composition. These powerful compounds, including carotenoids and tocopherols, lend their protective prowess to our cells, shielding them from the damaging effects of free radicals. Through their presence, ghee becomes not just a source of sustenance but also a guardian of our well-being.

The tale of ghee's nutritional prowess would be incomplete without acknowledging its lactose-free and casein-free nature. Through the process of clarification, these components are separated from the butterfat, making ghee a suitable option for those with lactose intolerance or dairy sensitivities. It becomes a source of nourishment that transcends dietary limitations, embracing all who seek its benefits.

Dear reader, as we unravel the intricate composition of ghee, we are reminded of the profound interplay between food and our well-being. Ghee, with its abundance of healthy fats, essential vitamins, gut-supportive compounds, and protective antioxidants, emerges as a nutritional powerhouse, nurturing us holistically.

In the next chapter, we shall venture into the realm of digestive health, exploring how ghee's unique properties contribute to the well-being of our digestive system. So, let us continue on this enriching journey, where emotions intertwine with nourishment, and the golden elixir continues to reveal its transformative secrets.

If you'd like to continue with the rest of the book or have any specific requests, please let me know!

Chapter 4: A Journey Within: Ghee and Digestive Wellness

In the intricate tapestry of our bodies, the digestive system weaves the threads of nourishment and vitality. It is within this sacred realm that ghee finds its true calling , a gentle healer, a soothing balm, and a guardian of digestive wellness. Let us embark on a journey into the depths of this remarkable synergy, where the golden elixir and our digestive system intertwine in perfect harmony.

As ghee graces our palates, it sets in motion a symphony of digestive support. The journey begins with the act of consumption, as the velvety richness of ghee coats the walls of the digestive tract with a tender embrace. It forms a protective barrier, shielding delicate tissues from irritation and inflammation, and paving the way for a seamless digestion.

Within the depths of ghee lies a treasure trove of butyric acid , a nurturing gift bestowed upon us. This precious fatty acid, derived from the fermentation of dietary fibers by gut bacteria, is not only present within ghee but is also produced by our own intestinal flora. As ghee makes its way through the digestive system, the butyric acid within harmonizes with the body's own supply, creating a nourishing environment for the cells lining the colon. It is a gentle healer, a source of comfort that fosters the well-being of our digestive sanctuary.

But the tale of ghee's digestive prowess does not end there. Its medium-chain fatty acids, easily absorbed and utilized by the body, provide a quick source of fuel and spare the digestive system unnecessary strain. In a world often marked by digestive woes, ghee emerges as a gentle companion, relieving the burden on the digestive system and allowing it to function with ease.

As the digestive journey unfolds, we encounter ghee's role in enhancing nutrient absorption. The presence of healthy fats in ghee aids in the absorption of fat-soluble vitamins, unlocking their full potential and delivering their nourishing benefits to every cell of our being. It is a testament to the synergistic dance between ghee and the digestive system, where optimal wellness is nurtured through their partnership.

But the healing power of ghee transcends mere physical nourishment , it reaches into the realm of emotions. As we partake in the golden elixir, we are invited to a journey of comfort and solace. The act of consuming ghee becomes an act of self-care, a moment of respite in a fast-paced world. It touches us on a deeper level, awakening the memories of simpler times, when a warm meal prepared with love was a balm for the soul.

Dear reader, as we immerse ourselves in the transformative alliance between ghee and digestive wellness, we bear witness to the intricate connections between our bodies and the nourishment we consume. Ghee, with its gentle healing properties, becomes a steadfast companion, supporting the delicate balance of our digestive system and nurturing our well-being on both physical and emotional levels.

In the upcoming chapter, we shall explore the diverse culinary applications of ghee, unraveling its versatility and embracing the art of flavor exploration. So, let us continue on this nourishing expedition, where emotions intertwine with culinary delight, and the golden elixir continues to enchant our senses.

If you'd like to continue with the rest of the book or have any specific requests, please let me know!

Chapter 5: A Symphony of Flavors: Culinary Magic with Ghee

In the realm of culinary artistry, ghee emerges as a maestro, conducting a symphony of flavors that dance upon our taste buds and resonate deep within our souls. It is a culinary treasure, a versatile ingredient that transcends boundaries and transforms every dish it graces. Let us embark on a journey into the world of culinary magic, where ghee becomes our guiding light, illuminating the path to unparalleled gastronomic experiences.

Within the realm of savory delights, ghee stands tall as a beacon of flavor enhancement. As it melts into a shimmering pool of golden goodness, it imparts a rich, nutty aroma that beckons us closer. With every sizzle and crackle, anticipation builds, and the kitchen becomes an arena of tantalizing possibilities.

Imagine a humble pan, its surface kissed by the golden touch of ghee. As ingredients are added, they are enveloped in a loving embrace, their flavors intensified and elevated to new heights. The gentle warmth of ghee coaxes out the inherent aromas, infusing the dish with a depth that captivates the senses. From vibrant curries to succulent stir-fries, ghee leaves its indelible mark, creating a symphony of flavors that resonates with every bite.

But the realm of ghee's culinary prowess extends far beyond savory delicacies. In the realm of baking, ghee becomes an enchanting muse, imparting a velvety richness and a delicate hint of nuttiness. It weaves its magic into flaky pastries, tender cakes, and golden-brown cookies, elevating each creation to a realm of pure delight. The touch of ghee transforms these treats into edible poetry, captivating hearts and palates alike.

And let us not forget the realm of simple pleasures , those moments when a dollop of ghee finds its way onto warm toast or steaming rice. The act of spreading ghee becomes a gesture of love, infusing each morsel with comfort and nostalgia. It is a reminder of the beauty in simplicity, where the true essence of ghee shines through, unadorned and pure.

Dear reader, as we immerse ourselves in the symphony of flavors woven by ghee, we are invited to embrace the art of culinary exploration. Ghee, with its transformative powers, becomes our guiding star, igniting our creativity and inviting us to embark on a gastronomic adventure. It is a testament to the profound connection between food and emotions, where a single ingredient can evoke memories, stir passions, and nourish the soul.

In the next chapter, we shall venture into the realm of self-care, exploring the ancient rituals and healing traditions associated with ghee. So, let us continue on this flavorful expedition, where emotions intertwine with culinary delight, and the golden elixir continues to weave its magic.

If you'd like to continue with the rest of the book or have any specific requests, please let me know!

Chapter 6: Embracing Self-Care: Ghee in Ancient Rituals and Healing Traditions

In the vast tapestry of human existence, self-care emerges as a sacred thread , a gentle reminder to nurture our bodies, minds, and spirits. Within this tapestry, ghee holds a special place, its golden radiance intertwined with ancient rituals and healing traditions that span across cultures and time. Let us embark on a journey of self-discovery, where the wisdom of the ages meets the transformative power of ghee.

From the dawn of civilization, ghee has been revered as more than just a culinary delight , it has been hailed as a symbol of purity, auspiciousness, and well-being. In ancient rituals, ghee played a central role, serving as an offering to the divine and a conduit for spiritual connection. Its luminous glow was believed to carry prayers and intentions to the heavens, bridging the gap between mortal and divine realms.

Beyond its spiritual significance, ghee has long been celebrated for its therapeutic properties. In Ayurvedic medicine, the ancient Indian system of healing, ghee holds a revered position as a carrier of medicinal herbs and a potent elixir in its own right. It is believed to balance the doshas, the elemental energies within the body, and promote overall wellness.

In the realm of skincare, ghee becomes a gentle ally, nourishing and rejuvenating the skin from within. Its natural emollient properties hydrate and soften the skin, leaving it supple and radiant. Through the ages, women and men have turned to ghee as a luxurious beauty treatment, an elixir of youth that transcends time.

But the realm of self-care encompasses more than just the physical , it delves into the realms of emotional well-being and nourishment of the soul. In the practices of meditation and mindfulness, ghee becomes a symbol of grounding and serenity. Its presence in rituals and offerings becomes a tangible representation of self-love and gratitude, a reminder to honor ourselves and cultivate inner peace.

Dear reader, as we immerse ourselves in the realm of self-care woven by ghee, we honor the wisdom of our ancestors and embrace the transformative power of ancient traditions. Ghee becomes a gentle guide, leading us on a path of holistic well-being, where body, mind, and spirit find harmony. It is a testament to the profound connection between rituals, healing, and the cultivation of our inner selves.

In the upcoming chapter, we shall explore the fusion of flavors and cultures, discovering how ghee transcends borders and becomes a unifying force in culinary exploration. So, let us continue on this nourishing expedition, where emotions intertwine with ancient wisdom, and the golden elixir continues to illuminate our path.

If you'd like to continue with the rest of the book or have any specific requests, please let me know!

Chapter 7: Fusion of Flavors: Ghee as a Unifying Force in Culinary Exploration

In the vibrant tapestry of global cuisine, flavors and traditions interweave, creating a harmonious symphony that transcends borders and unites cultures. At the heart of this culinary fusion stands ghee , an ambassador of richness and depth, a unifying force that bridges the gap between diverse culinary traditions. Let us embark on a journey of flavor exploration, where ghee becomes the catalyst for culinary harmony and cultural exchange.

As we traverse continents, our taste buds embark on an adventure, experiencing the myriad flavors that ghee infuses into each dish it encounters. In the bustling streets of India, ghee dances with aromatic spices, giving birth to curries that transport us to a land of bold flavors and vibrant hues. Its golden essence harmonizes with cumin, coriander, turmeric, and a myriad of other spices, creating a symphony of taste that tantalizes and satisfies.

In the enchanting landscapes of the Mediterranean, ghee mingles with sun-ripened olives, fragrant herbs, and succulent vegetables. It becomes the essence that unites Greek moussaka, Turkish pilaf, and Moroccan tagines, infusing each dish with a richness that transcends cultural boundaries. Ghee embraces the flavors of the Mediterranean, forging a connection between lands and inviting us to savor the diversity of the region.

Across the vast expanse of Asia, ghee becomes a common thread that weaves together the culinary traditions of countless nations. In the fiery stir-fries of China, the aromatic curries of Thailand, and the delicate sushi rolls of Japan, ghee leaves its mark, adding a layer of complexity and depth to every bite. It transcends borders, embracing the nuances of Asian cuisine, and revealing the power of culinary fusion.

In the melting pot of the Americas, ghee finds its place, adapting and blending into the diverse tapestry of flavors. It lends its richness to Mexican salsas, Colombian arepas, and Brazilian feijoadas, embracing the vibrancy of

Latin American cuisine. Ghee becomes an agent of integration, a unifying force that celebrates the melting pot of cultures found within the continent.

Dear reader, as we embark on this culinary exploration, we witness the power of ghee to transcend borders and unite cultures through the medium of flavor. It becomes an ambassador of harmony, bridging the gaps between diverse culinary traditions and fostering a sense of interconnectedness. Through the fusion of flavors, we celebrate the beauty of diversity and embrace the richness that comes from cultural exchange.

In the next chapter, we shall delve into the realm of ghee's culinary versatility, exploring its uses in both traditional and contemporary recipes. So, let us continue on this flavorful expedition, where emotions intertwine with culinary discovery, and the golden elixir continues to expand our culinary horizons.

If you'd like to continue with the rest of the book or have any specific requests, please let me know!

Chapter 8: A Culinary Kaleidoscope: Ghee's Versatility in Traditional and Contemporary Recipes

In the ever-evolving world of culinary delights, ghee emerges as a versatile muse, inspiring chefs and home cooks alike to explore new frontiers of flavor and creativity. Its golden presence graces both traditional recipes handed down through generations and contemporary culinary creations that push the boundaries of taste. Let us embark on a culinary kaleidoscope, where ghee's versatility shines brightly, illuminating the realm of both time-honored classics and innovative dishes.

In the realm of traditional recipes, ghee takes on the role of an honored companion, imparting its unique richness and depth to beloved dishes. Picture a pot of simmering dal, its aroma filling the air with warmth and comfort. As ghee is added, it elevates the humble lentils to new heights, lending a velvety texture and a buttery essence that evokes memories of home-cooked meals and gatherings with loved ones.

Across continents and cultures, ghee leaves its mark on traditional bread-making techniques. In the Indian subcontinent, it is the key to creating fluffy naan and buttery parathas that melt in your mouth. In France, ghee finds its counterpart in the delicate layers of puff pastry, creating the golden, flaky perfection of a croissant. Ghee becomes the secret ingredient that transforms these breads into works of edible art, each bite evoking a symphony of textures and flavors.

But ghee's versatility extends far beyond the boundaries of tradition. In the realm of contemporary cuisine, it becomes a canvas for culinary experimentation, allowing chefs to push the boundaries of taste and create innovative dishes that challenge our palates. From ghee-infused desserts that blend sweet and savory to unique flavor combinations in savory dishes, ghee becomes a vehicle for culinary exploration, adding a touch of indulgence and complexity.

Imagine a velvety chocolate cake, its richness amplified by the addition of ghee. As it melts on the tongue, the flavors dance , a symphony of decadence that transports us to a realm of pure bliss. In the realm of savory delights, ghee finds its place in unexpected combinations , a drizzle of spiced ghee over roasted vegetables, a dollop of infused ghee on a grilled steak. Each bite becomes an adventure, a tantalizing exploration of flavors that surprises and delights.

Dear reader, as we delve into the realm of ghee's versatility, we witness its ability to honor tradition while embracing innovation. It becomes a companion in the kitchen, inspiring us to infuse our creations with richness and depth. Through both time-honored recipes and contemporary culinary marvels, ghee continues to spark our imagination and nourish our senses.

In the upcoming chapter, we shall uncover the secrets of ghee's shelf life and storage, ensuring that this golden elixir remains a cherished ally in our culinary endeavors. So, let us continue on this flavorful expedition, where emotions intertwine with culinary mastery, and the golden elixir continues to ignite our passion for cooking.

If you'd like to continue with the rest of the book or have any specific requests, please let me know!

Chapter 9: Preserving Liquid Gold: Ghee's Shelf Life and Storage Secrets

In the realm of culinary alchemy, ghee stands as a testament to the art of preservation , a golden elixir that withstands the tests of time, preserving its rich flavor and nourishing properties. As guardians of this liquid gold, we embark on a journey of knowledge, exploring the secrets to ghee's extended shelf life and the art of proper storage. Let us delve into the realm of preservation, where emotions intertwine with the preciousness of this culinary treasure.

Like a time capsule of flavors, ghee possesses an exceptional shelf life that sets it apart from other ingredients. Through the process of clarification, the milk solids are removed, leaving behind a pure, clarified butter that can be stored for extended periods. This removal of moisture and impurities contributes to ghee's longevity, allowing it to retain its rich flavor and nutritional benefits for months, if not years.

The key to preserving ghee lies in ensuring its purity and protection from external elements. To begin, it is crucial to start with quality ingredients , unsalted butter made from the milk of grass-fed cows is the foundation for exceptional ghee. This butter is simmered slowly, allowing the milk solids to separate and the water content to evaporate, resulting in a clarified liquid gold.

Once the ghee is prepared, proper storage becomes paramount. The ideal conditions for preserving ghee include a cool, dry, and dark environment. Airtight containers made of glass or stainless steel are excellent choices, as they protect the ghee from exposure to air, light, and moisture. These containers serve as guardians, shielding the golden elixir and ensuring its longevity.

As we gaze upon our collection of ghee, each jar becomes a vessel of memories , a reflection of culinary journeys, cherished moments, and flavors that have touched our hearts. With each opening, we release a burst of aroma , a reminder of the journey ghee has taken, from its creation to our very fingertips. It is a sensory experience that ignites emotions and fuels our culinary passion.

Dear reader, as we embrace the art of preserving ghee, we honor its preciousness and the significance it holds in our culinary repertoire. Through proper storage and mindful care, we extend the lifespan of this liquid gold, ensuring that its flavor and nourishing qualities remain intact. In doing so, we become the custodians of ghee's legacy, embracing the responsibility to protect and savor its essence.

In the following chapter, we shall explore the myriad health benefits of ghee, delving into the ways it nourishes our bodies and supports our well-being. So, let us continue on this flavorful expedition, where emotions intertwine with the preservation of culinary treasures, and the golden elixir continues to grace our tables.

If you'd like to continue with the rest of the book or have any specific requests, please let me know!

Chapter 10: Nourishing Body and Soul: Ghee's Bountiful Health Benefits

In the realm of culinary enchantment, ghee emerges not only as a delightful addition to our dishes but also as a source of nourishment for both body and soul. As we explore the health benefits of ghee, we unravel a tapestry woven with care, wisdom, and the transformative power of this golden elixir. Let us embark on a journey of well-being, where emotions intertwine with the bountiful gifts that ghee bestows upon us.

Ghee, revered for centuries as a sacred substance, carries within it a multitude of health benefits that span across mind, body, and spirit. As we consume this radiant elixir, its inherent qualities nurture our physical well-being and ignite a sense of vitality within.

At the core of ghee's health benefits lies its unique composition. With its high smoke point and absence of lactose and casein, ghee becomes a friendly companion for those with lactose sensitivities. Its rich source of medium-chain fatty acids, including butyric acid, supports digestive health, soothes inflammation, and aids in nutrient absorption. Ghee becomes a gentle ally, providing comfort and nourishment to those seeking a balanced and harmonious digestive system.

As we delve deeper into the realm of ghee, we uncover its potential to promote heart health. Contrary to what intuition may suggest, ghee possesses properties that may aid in maintaining healthy cholesterol levels. Its composition of saturated fats, when consumed in moderation, can contribute to a healthy lipid profile, ensuring the well-being of our cardiovascular system.

But ghee's gifts extend far beyond the physical realm. In the ancient traditions of Ayurveda, ghee is hailed as a tonic for the mind and spirit. Its nourishing qualities are believed to enhance memory, sharpen intellect, and promote mental clarity. It becomes a sacred vessel, carrying within it the potential to kindle the flame of creativity and ignite the spark of inspiration within us.

In the realm of self-care, ghee takes on the role of a gentle guardian, nurturing our skin and radiating a youthful glow. Its moisturizing properties penetrate deep into the layers of our skin, leaving it soft, supple, and rejuvenated. As we embrace ghee's touch, we indulge in a ritual of self-love, honoring our bodies and cherishing the essence of our being.

Dear reader, as we immerse ourselves in the bountiful health benefits of ghee, we embrace the power of this golden elixir to nourish not only our bodies but also our souls. It becomes a conduit for holistic well-being, intertwining the realms of physical vitality, mental clarity, and emotional serenity. With each spoonful, we savor the gift of wellness, savoring the profound connection between ghee and our journey towards optimal health.

In the upcoming chapter, we shall explore the culinary magic of ghee in more detail, unveiling the art of incorporating ghee into a variety of dishes and recipes. So, let us continue on this flavorful expedition, where emotions intertwine with the nourishing qualities of ghee, and the golden elixir continues to grace our lives.

If you'd like to continue with the rest of the book or have any specific requests, please let me know!

Chapter 11: The Culinary Alchemy: Ghee's Magic in Every Bite

In the realm of culinary enchantment, ghee takes center stage as a mystical ingredient , a golden elixir that possesses the power to transform ordinary dishes into extraordinary culinary creations. As we dive into the depths of ghee's culinary alchemy, we uncover the magic that unfolds with every delectable bite. Join me on this journey of flavor and wonder, where emotions intertwine with the enchanting power of ghee.

Imagine a sizzling pan, where a dollop of ghee meets the heat with a gentle hiss. Instantly, an aroma fills the air , a symphony of nutty richness that awakens the senses. As ghee embraces the ingredients, it weaves its magic, infusing each morsel with a layer of complexity and depth. Every bite becomes a revelation , a sensory experience that transcends mere sustenance, captivating our taste buds and stirring our emotions.

In the realm of sautÃ©s and stir-fries, ghee dances with vibrant vegetables, tender meats, and fragrant spices. It coats each ingredient, unlocking their flavors and creating a harmonious melody that sings on our palates. As we take that first mouthful, a burst of delight envelops us , an orchestra of taste that brings joy and nourishment, weaving a tapestry of emotions that elevates the act of eating to an art form.

But ghee's magic extends beyond the realms of savory delights. In the realm of baking, it becomes a secret weapon , a culinary spell that transforms doughs and batters into works of edible art. Picture a flaky pie crust, its layers delicately intertwined, beckoning us to savor its buttery embrace. Ghee, with its unrivaled richness, takes center stage, infusing each bite with a velvety texture that melts in our mouths, evoking a symphony of pleasure and satisfaction.

As we explore the world of desserts, ghee reveals its ability to transcend boundaries and blend flavors with finesse. It becomes the bridge that unites sweet and savory, allowing us to create confections that surprise and delight. From ghee-infused caramel drizzled over desserts to the delicate balance it brings to spiced sweets, ghee adds a touch of magic, igniting our senses and transporting us to a realm of sweet enchantment.

Dear reader, as we savor the culinary alchemy of ghee, we witness its transformative power in every bite. It becomes the spark that ignites our creativity, the ingredient that elevates our dishes from ordinary to extraordinary. Through its magic, we connect with the essence of food , the ability to nourish not only our bodies but also our souls, stirring emotions and creating memories that linger long after the last morsel has been enjoyed.

In the following chapter, we shall delve into the art of incorporating ghee into everyday cooking, providing you with practical tips and recipes that celebrate the versatility of this golden elixir. So, let us continue on this flavorful expedition, where emotions intertwine with the mystical nature of ghee, and the culinary alchemy continues to ignite our passion for the culinary arts.

If you'd like to continue with the rest of the book or have any specific requests, please let me know!

Chapter 12: Ghee in Everyday Cooking: A Symphony of Flavors

In the symphony of everyday cooking, ghee takes its place as a conductor, orchestrating a medley of flavors that dance upon our palates. As we explore the art of incorporating ghee into our daily culinary endeavors, we unlock a world of possibilities , a realm where simplicity meets sophistication, and emotions intertwine with the harmonious balance of flavors. Join me on this culinary symphony, where ghee takes center stage, conducting a masterpiece in every dish.

In the realm of breakfast, ghee becomes a morning serenade , a soothing melody that begins our day on a flavorful note. Imagine a slice of warm toast, lightly adorned with a spread of ghee. With each bite, the buttery richness envelops us, evoking a sense of comfort and contentment. Ghee becomes the conductor that sets the stage, infusing our breakfast with a symphony of flavors that awaken our senses and prepare us for the day ahead.

As we progress to the realm of soups and stews, ghee adds depth and complexity to humble ingredients, transforming them into culinary symphonies. Picture a pot of aromatic tomato soup, simmering gently on the stovetop. With a touch of ghee, the flavors intensify , a harmony of sweetness and acidity that lingers on our tongues. Ghee becomes the maestro, conducting the ensemble of ingredients, ensuring that each spoonful is a journey of flavor and emotion.

In the realm of side dishes, ghee lends its golden touch to elevate the simplest of ingredients into culinary masterpieces. Take roasted vegetables, for example. As they roast in the oven, ghee envelops them with a luscious coat, caramelizing and intensifying their natural sweetness. Each bite becomes a celebration of flavors , a symphony of textures and tastes that dance upon our palates, leaving us yearning for more.

But ghee's influence doesn't stop there. In the realm of indulgent desserts, it becomes the secret ingredient that enhances the symphony of sweetness. Imagine a warm apple crumble, fresh out of the oven. As we take that first bite, the buttery essence of ghee melds with the sweet apples, creating a heavenly fusion of flavors that stirs our emotions and brings joy to our hearts. Ghee becomes the virtuoso, infusing our desserts with a richness and complexity that leaves a lasting impression.

Dear reader, as we embrace the art of incorporating ghee into everyday cooking, we discover its ability to elevate even the simplest of dishes. It becomes the conductor of flavor , a symphony of taste that delights our palates and nourishes our souls. Through the harmonious balance of ingredients and the golden touch of ghee, we embark on a culinary journey that transcends the ordinary, creating moments of joy and connection through the transformative power of food.

In the upcoming chapter, we shall explore the cultural significance of ghee, unraveling its presence in traditional cuisines and the role it plays in celebrations and rituals. So, let us continue on this flavorful expedition, where emotions intertwine with the symphony of ghee in everyday cooking, and the culinary arts continue to captivate our hearts.

If you'd like to continue with the rest of the book or have any specific requests, please let me know!

Chapter 13: Ghee in Cultural Cuisine: A Tapestry of Tradition and Flavor

In the tapestry of cultural cuisine, ghee weaves its way through the rich fabric of tradition and flavor, leaving behind a trail of history and nostalgia. As we delve into the cultural significance of ghee, we unravel a story of culinary heritage , a tale that connects us to our roots, stirs our emotions, and evokes a sense of belonging. Join me on this journey through time and taste, where ghee becomes a symbol of cultural identity and a conduit for preserving tradition.

In the realm of Indian cuisine, ghee reigns supreme , a culinary emblem that has stood the test of time. It holds a sacred place in Indian households, transcending mere ingredients to become a symbol of love and nourishment. Passed down through generations, ghee carries the wisdom of ancestors, infusing every dish with their presence and a sense of familial connection. It becomes the thread that binds families together, bridging the gap between past and present.

From the vibrant curries of North India to the delicate flavors of South Indian cuisine, ghee plays a pivotal role, lending its distinctive richness and aroma to each dish. Picture a bowl of creamy dal, the golden ghee pooling on its surface , a visual representation of comfort and sustenance. With each spoonful, we savor the essence of tradition , a taste that transports us to a time when recipes were whispered from grandmother to grandchild, nurturing not only our bodies but also our spirits.

Beyond Indian cuisine, ghee finds its place in a multitude of cultural traditions, each with its unique rituals and flavors. In Middle Eastern cuisine, ghee takes the form of clarified butter , a symbol of hospitality and abundance.

It graces dishes like basbousa and baklava, infusing them with a velvety richness that captivates our taste buds and creates a sense of warmth and togetherness. With each bite, we experience a taste of the region's history and the spirit of generosity that defines its culinary culture.

In the melting pot of global gastronomy, ghee finds its way into diverse cuisines, adapting and harmonizing with different flavors and cooking techniques. From the flaky layers of French pastries enriched with ghee to the fragrant biryanis of Southeast Asia infused with its nutty aroma, ghee becomes a universal language , a bridge that connects cultures and unites us through the universal pleasure of food.

Dear reader, as we explore the cultural significance of ghee, we immerse ourselves in a world of tradition, flavor, and connection. It becomes a vessel for preserving heritage and celebrating diversity , a thread that weaves through the fabric of cultural cuisine, nurturing our souls and reminding us of our shared humanity. Through the essence of ghee, we honor the past, savor the present, and pave the way for a future where culinary traditions continue to inspire and unite.

In the final chapter of our journey, we shall reflect on the profound impact of ghee, both in the kitchen and in our lives. We will explore the transformative power of food and the emotional resonance it holds. So, let us continue on this flavorful expedition, where emotions intertwine with the cultural significance of ghee, and the culinary tapestry continues to unfold.

If you'd like to continue with the conclusion or have any specific requests, please let me know!

Chapter 14: The Transformative Power of Ghee: Nourishing Body and Soul

In the realm of culinary enchantment, ghee emerges as more than just an ingredient , it becomes a transformative elixir that nourishes not only our bodies but also our souls. As we reflect on the profound impact of ghee, we uncover its ability to create moments of joy, connection, and healing. Join me on this final chapter of our journey, where we explore the transformative power of ghee, and how it leaves an indelible mark on our lives.

In the kitchen, ghee serves as a catalyst for creativity , a spark that ignites our passion for cooking and encourages experimentation. As we drizzle ghee over roasted vegetables, stir it into curries, or fold it into baked goods, we embark on a journey of culinary exploration. It empowers us to infuse every dish with a touch of magic, to infuse every meal with love and care, turning the act of cooking into an expression of artistry and self-discovery.

But ghee's transformative power extends far beyond the boundaries of the kitchen. It becomes a vehicle for connection , a medium through which we express our love and affection for others. Picture a family gathered around the dinner table, sharing a meal enriched with the goodness of ghee. With each bite, they share more than just food; they share laughter, stories, and a sense of togetherness that nourishes their souls. Ghee becomes the invisible thread that binds them, fostering a sense of belonging and unity.

In times of celebration and ritual, ghee takes on a sacred role , a symbol of purity and offering. From the glowing diyas of Diwali to the festive sweets prepared for Eid, ghee plays a central part in these cherished traditions. Its presence elevates these occasions, infusing them with a sense of reverence and spirituality. Through the act of preparing and sharing ghee-laden delicacies, we pay homage to our cultural heritage and strengthen the ties that bind us to our roots.

Moreover, ghee carries the power of healing , an ancient wisdom that has been revered for centuries. In Ayurveda, ghee is regarded as a medicinal elixir, believed to have nourishing and rejuvenating properties. When consumed mindfully and in moderation, it can promote balance and well-being, soothing both body and mind. As we partake in dishes made with ghee, we invite healing into our lives, nurturing ourselves from the inside out.

Dear reader, as we come to the end of our journey through the world of ghee, we find that it has touched our lives in profound ways. It has sparked our creativity, strengthened our connections, celebrated our traditions, and nurtured our well-being. Through the transformative power of ghee, we have discovered that food is more than just sustenance , it is an art, a language, and a conduit for emotions.

So, let us carry this newfound appreciation for ghee into our daily lives, infusing our meals with love and intention. Let us cherish the moments spent with loved ones around the table, where ghee becomes the medium for creating memories that last a lifetime.

And as we continue to explore the vast world of culinary enchantment, let us always remember the magic of ghee , a golden elixir that nourishes not only our bodies but also our hearts and souls.

With this chapter, we conclude our flavorful journey through the world of ghee and its transformative power. If you have any additional requests or topics you'd like to explore further, please let me know!

Chapter 15: A Farewell to Ghee: Embracing the Legacy

As we bid farewell to our beloved companion in the culinary symphony, ghee, we are filled with bittersweet emotions , a mingling of gratitude and nostalgia. Throughout our journey, it has been more than just an ingredient , it has been a faithful companion, an artistic muse, and a conduit for emotions that have enriched our lives. In this final chapter, we reflect on the legacy of ghee and how its essence will forever linger in our hearts and kitchens.

In the kitchen, ghee's legacy endures through the recipes passed down from one generation to the next. These culinary heirlooms carry the imprints of loved ones , the aroma of their kitchens, the rhythm of their cooking, and the joy they felt in sharing meals with family and friends. As we recreate these cherished dishes, we imbue them with the same love and care that have been woven into their very fabric, honoring the legacy of those who came before us.

Beyond the realm of family traditions, ghee's legacy extends into the broader tapestry of culture and community. It remains an essential ingredient in the kitchens of countless homes, each with its unique flavors and stories. Its versatility allows it to adapt to various cuisines, embracing diversity and fostering a sense of unity. It connects us to a global family of food enthusiasts , a community bound by the love of flavors and the joy of cooking.

In the face of modern culinary trends and convenience, ghee stands as a timeless symbol of tradition and authenticity. Its enduring presence serves as a reminder that the simplest of ingredients can hold the power to transform and elevate our culinary experiences. As we continue to incorporate ghee into our cooking, we pay homage to the culinary wisdom of our ancestors and the enduring significance of tradition in our rapidly changing world.

Moreover, the legacy of ghee is a testament to the emotional resonance of food. It has the power to evoke memories, to transport us back in time, and to create new moments of connection. As we savor dishes infused with the golden touch of ghee, we experience the magic of taste , an experience that transcends the boundaries of language and culture, speaking directly to our hearts.

As we bid farewell to this journey through the world of ghee, we carry its legacy with us , like a treasure chest filled with culinary wonders. Let us continue to explore the realms of flavor, creativity, and connection, infusing our meals with the same passion and emotion that ghee has inspired within us. With every dish we prepare, we celebrate the artistry of cooking, the joy of sharing, and the legacy of flavors that have shaped our lives.

Dear reader, it is with a mix of happiness and wistfulness that we embrace the legacy of ghee , a legacy that will forever reside in our kitchens and hearts. Let us honor this golden elixir by savoring its essence in every dish we create and by cherishing the memories it has kindled along the way. As we move forward on our culinary journey, may the legacy of ghee continue to guide us, inspire us, and remind us of the enduring magic of food.

With this final chapter, our journey through the world of ghee comes to a close. I hope you have enjoyed this flavorful expedition, and if you have any more requests or topics you'd like

to explore, please feel free to let me
know!

Printed in Great Britain
by Amazon

32150408R00042